The Home Health Care Industry in the U.S.: UNTOLD REALITIES

Delavil Lekunze

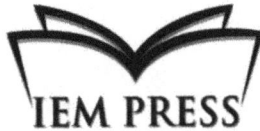

IEM PRESS

PO Box 831001, Richardson, TX 75080

A Subsidiary of IEM APPROACH

IEM PRESS (PO Box 831001, Richardson, TX 75080) functions only as book publisher. As such, the ultimate design, content, editorial accuracy, and views expressed or implied in this work are those of the author. No part of this publication may be reproduced, stored in a retrieval system, or transmitted in any way—electronic, mechanical, photocopy, recording, or other-wise—without the copyright holder's prior permission, except as provided by USA copyright law.

ISBN 13: 978-1-63603-021-0

Library of Congress Catalog Card Number : 2021900579

CONTENTS

ACKNOWLEDGEMENTS

I am grateful to all who made useful contributions to this work.

Firstly, to the caregivers, their clients, staff and owners of various home healthcare companies, physicians, therapists, and social workers, most of whom answered my questions without hesitating;

Ms. Belinda Asare, whose courage, encouragement, and challenging rise to become a homecare company owner in the U.S. gave push to this work;

Mr. Joel of KJOE Art, blessed with outstanding creative talents, who dedicated time and much effort to design the book's cover;

Pastor Prince Bright for his unwavering spiritual backing and prayers;

Mr. Sylvanus Ano for proofreading and editing;

My sister Nama and brother Peter, for proofreading, making useful proposals, and for his retouch of the title;

Mr. Jesma Bakowi and Mr. Taphe Jonathan for suggestions that helped improve the work;

Other contributors, editors, and proofreaders who cannot all be mentioned here.

DEDICATION

This work is dedicated to my family, my parents: Daniel Ketoma Lekunze, in honour of his integrity and genuine care for people; my mother, Regina Nanzi for the same reasons. She is the most hardworking and loving, caring mother I have ever seen, always catering for all children like hers. I learn big lessons about caring for others from her.

To my late grandmother Susan Nagang, who passed over the successor Stool to me, to keep afloat all that she cherished; and my late grandfather his Majesty Lekunze Nembongwe. He lived a historic, glorious life that will positively impact generations for a long time. A man whose demonstration of wisdom in family management, peace building, and compassion for his numerous children and those of an entire clan earned him much respect from his people.

Also dedicated to my late maternal grandparents, ma Natsi and Ketuama.

PREFACE

A less complex approach to anything we do will make our lives much easier to manage and more joy filled. This happens when we follow the Creator's basic rules for a good life, which results in sound health and the world being a better place for all. Do unto others as you would want them do to you, love your neighbor as yourself, obey and honor your father and mother are the rules that, if respected, will turn our small worlds toward fulfilling paths. When these values animate you, you develop a healthy mindset, which begets a healthy body and a healthy society. Undermining them is causing all the disasters plaguing us - wars, human rights violations, genocide, torture, power abuse, murder, family disintegration, neglect of close relations, especially our parents who are pillars of our existence.

In Western societies, social services and the home healthcare industry come in to fill the loopholes left in our call to duty toward loved ones. Research is proving that even if all other industries here should die someday, those of home healthcare will survive due to rapid progress in scientific discoveries that lengthen the lives of humans.

When this caught my attention, I decided to dig further into the innerworkings of this booming industry. While doing that, rising complaints and bitter criticisms about its functioning from those in its network pushed me to uncover untold realities in the sector.

This book presents a glimpse of the cacophony, joys and abuses in the industry, which will over-whelm you as you read on.

During extensive investigations, I talked to vari-ous parties offering services in home healthcare - company managers and owners, social work-ers, physical therapists, physicians, nurses, and hundreds of caregivers and their clients. It was exciting and at the same time heartbreaking listening to their stories. These caregivers (home health aides) are the backbone of the industry, and without them, it can easily collapse. Yet the majority of them are so underestimated, underpaid and abused almost all the time. Without them, most of our elderly and younger ones taken care of by home-care services would find their lives gone at a snap. There is a lot to blow your mind as you read their stories and those of clients they care for here, serving a big lesson, especially to readers who intend to live in the United States and Europe all their lives.

An x-ray of the industry in this book opens our eyes to some minor but crucial issues that we probably overlook, ignorant of dangerous negative effects that they can have on us, our health, and family bonding. As you get to know about them, your lifestyle, treatment of your parents, and the way you manage your possessions may never be the same again.

INTRODUCTION

The health complications that we face as we grow older depend on the lifestyles we choose. Avoiding excesses in most things we do, especially in food consumption and eating the right way, acting with decency and spiritual uprightness are major escape routes from illnesses that hold many people hostage, mostly in their golden years.

If you live in the U.S. or in any other western country and neglect these, then be ready for some battles in later stages of your life, which we will be revealing here. When that time comes, depending on the kind of insurance you have or what your pocket can afford, arrangements are made for a chain of health professionals to attend to you regularly. They will come knocking at your door or calling on the phone to book appointments for endless consultations.

The physical therapists, caregivers (home health aides), social workers, doctors, nurses, chiropractors, and all kinds of specialists will be connected to you. Most elderly people would tell you how overwhelming that can be sometimes, looking like an invasion of everything about them. Often the decision may not be theirs but that of their social worker, caretaker, family, confidant, or their power of attorney.

In a comment, 81 year old Edna says, "I keep asking what this physical therapist comes to my house thrice a week to do. He will sit here, raise my hand, and swing it left and right for twenty minutes. Then sends a check of $580 at end of month for me to pay. Whoever made such arrangement with him is a puzzle because my caregiver could do better than what he drives for two hours to come do here. Even my daughter can do that."

Like many of her age do, Edna complains because she does not understand the techniques applied to those gentle swings of the physical therapist, which cannot be mastered by those not trained for the job. This is just an example of the repulsion many clients express toward some home health services that they consider unnecessary but are imposed on them. It is often because no one took time to explain their importance and the intricacies in their functioning systems, to the patient.

Home care providers are multiplying fast as the industry keeps rising to the top in the healthcare sector. Research by Ibis World (1) shows an average industry growth of 4.3% in 2015-2020. Their report highlights how home care saves patients billions of dollars every year when treated in their own homes instead of in hospitals. An aging population, the prevalence of chronic diseases, growing physician acceptance of home care, medical advancements, and a movement toward cost-efficient treatment options from public and private payers have all fostered industry growth.

Population, increasing interest in home healthcare, and expanded access to Medicare and Medicaid under the Patient Protection and Affordable Care Act (PPACA) are influencing the growth, according to Ibis World. Its findings showed the following for 2014-2019.

Home Care Providers:

- Market size: $94 billion

- Number of businesses: 398,329

- Employment: 1,956,690

Companies in this industry primarily provide medical or non-medical services in the home. They include skilled nursing care, personal care, homemaker services, physical therapy, and medical social service. Others are in-home hospice care, traditional home healthcare, personal services, home therapy services, companion services, twenty-four-hour home care, in-home occupational and vocational therapy, speech therapy, and in-home dietary and nutritional services.

As we explore different chapters of this book, you will discover volumes about the world of home health care in Western societies, particularly in America. What is presented here will help get you prepared for whatever awaits you in their spider's web, when the time comes.

Even as the industry is well regulated with watch-dogs overseeing their practices, it is still packed full of problems.

Information for this work was gathered in assisted living communities, senior centers in the U.S., and from interviews with home health aides, manag-ers and owners of companies in the sector. Their clients and those involved in the chain (nurses, doctors, social workers, attorneys, physical thera-pists, insurers, case managers, powers of attorney, family relations, nutritionists etc.) were also inter-viewed.

These are the people who will stream in and out of your home quarterly or weekly, depending on your needs. The more complex your situation, the more frequent their visits will be. Unfortunately, many people are often not ready for this until that "magi-cal" hour of uncertainty strikes, reserving doom or gloom for them, following the choices they make.

INTRODUCTION
End Note

(1) *ibisworld.com: Home Care Providers Industry Research – Market Research, June, 2020).*

https://www.ibisworld.com/united-states/ market-research-reports/home-care-providers-industry/

ONE

COVID-19 WOES: CRUSHED BY THE NIGHTMARE

The monster pandemic took the world by storm. No alarm bells sounded before its arrival. Everyone was shocked, and shock has killed many just as the disease has done. Sandy, the most outspoken of all the caregivers interviewed for this work, went through near hell during the COVID-19 outbreak, and her enlightening words and experiences are touching.

SANDY'S STORY

Prrrmmm. There goes my phone ringing. It's my boss, Audrey. "Sandy, please, please, can you help out? We are excessively overwhelmed. I'm beyond confused. We can't leave our clients die in their homes. Many of our employees are adamant in refusing to go to work."

"Of course they shouldn't," I snap. "What do you expect? It's a state order for all to stay indoors. You know they will be fining me if I am outside at a certain hour, $5,000 plus a prison term, I hear."

"Not for workers like you," My Voice Quivers.

"Even if not for employees like me, I'm going nowhere," I grumble. That's the beauty of this job. You choosing to work when and where you want. Does she mean she didn't hear? Did Audrey not hear the spokesman of New York's Home Care Association Roger Noyes say, "It's a hair-on-fire crisis"?

I start reflecting on how much I have sacrificed for years caring for these white folk who hardly ever appreciate me but keep seeking ways to exterminate my people. I just read a series of ugly stories about the mystical COVID filth pointing to that. One story reports how they created the virus in a lab with their first target being Africans. And the other report warns against their vaccines, some of which in the past made millions of our children handicapped and our women sterile.

With all that I am learning from these stories, Ms. Audrey Golberg can have the audacity to call me to go to work for her white mother? To New York of all places? Where more than 100 people died just yesterday and deaths are still rising by the day and close to 30,000 in the past ten weeks? No way! She wants to say she hasn't read the stories when the social media is awash with them?

Some of these hair-raising reports are sending us Africans into hysteria as we can clearly see the degree of hatred these people exude toward us. See what is going on in China with my people. Expelled from their homes and hotels and dumped on the streets, accused of being those transmitting COVID-19 in that country, when we hear it was hatched in a lab in the same China. At the same time, you can see millions of Chinese and white folks roaming our streets and villages in Africa unperturbed. How foolish have we become? First time fool, you are forgiven. Second time fool, expect no ounce of forgiveness.

No, no, no, I am not going to cater for them in the name of kindness or home health aide (HHA) anymore. I have to quit the profession. So much anger is brewing in me that I fear I won't treat any of them with the genuine love, warmth, and enthusiasm that I used to have for these clients. I have decided to stay home for as long as the government has decreed, like all my neighbors are doing. It's all about my life, the lives of my sisters and brothers. Here we are, helping their parents, yet what most of them do is try to delete us from the globe.

Prrrrrrrrmmm again. "Please, Sandy, help, help," Audrey cuts in, panicking. "Most of our clients are in danger. We cannot abandon them. Looks like the other aides even fear touching their phones as much as they dread COVID. They aren't picking up my calls, and the few who do are screaming "no". I know you and some others still have a heart, please, please. Wherever you may be, I will send an Uber to pick you up."

This is the same Audrey who has always treated me like a nobody in the company now on her knees virtually crying for help. Yes, crying for help because if something happens to these clients, she will be held responsible and sued for neglect. "May that happen so they can spend all that money that they have been stealing from us, the aides," I murmur. Now I who was a nonentity have suddenly become savior, not only for her but also for her company.

I thought I should tell her to call all those white-skinned colleagues of mine to whom they granted all the favors. Paying them $17/hour and me $11/hour, giving them clients with whole legs while giving me amputees. I thought I could get out there to help any other agency in this America, not those of Audrey, Getty, Eleanor or Virginia, the devils who had got me through decimating flame when I worked with them in those awfully discriminating agencies.

Prrrrrrrrrrrrrrrmmm. "Sandy, I am waiting. Please let me know what you decide as soon as possible, sweetheart," she says, this time on voice-mail.

"Who is deciding what, forget it, damn you," Sandy grumbles.

For two days I can't sleep as I ruminate over this. I am next door to New York. In the news, they say dark clouds are hovering over the city. I always hated the Western media with their fake news, as President Trump slams them, and hardly ever watch them, especially as all they often report about my country and continent is filth, filth, filth. Even if we have puddles, which their countries also have, we have sunny facets that the world greatly admires when they discover them. But they never want to let people know.

Audrey doesn't have to bother me about anything now even, as I am still mourning the loss of parents of my friends Bridget in a senseless war. Since covid came, I don't think about it as much as I think about the ongoing genocide in her beautiful country called Southern Cameroons/Ambazonia for four years now - my one-time dream destination because of its good-natured people and exotic splendor. Yet none of these international media houses here is reporting about it. We see how the people weep every day. They have sent out thousands of reports and some of the most gruesome images of dehumanization of God's innocent creations. These pictures are not only splattered all over social media but have also been flooding the desks of power brokers at the United Nations, the European Union, CNN, BBC, plus hundreds more for four years. Still no concrete response, no detailed investigative report by any of them. Those desks are flooded because some of them have a hand in the genocide and possess internationally defined instruments set up by all the nations on earth to stop it. For me the genocide is even worst than covid19 in that country. I should now instead be thinking of how to help victims of such dehumanization, not Audrey and her cohorts.

Those great international institutions under the United Nations (U.N.) had all vowed that the 1994 Rwanda genocide was never to be repeated in this world. So what's happening? There has hardly been any reaction from them or coverage from influential international media houses. The mayhem, rapes, head cutting, burning down of more than four hundred villages, killing of over 20,0000 Ambazonians, one million internally displaced persons, and 200,000 plus as refugees in neighboring countries have been near non-events to them. But suddenly a coup d'état in Mali,

Africa, that occurred just last month in August is on the agenda of the upcoming U.N. General Assembly this September 2020, I hear. And this is the very place where Audrey's father works and sits watching with his colleagues, saying nothing on a situation which they could have saved from degenerating on the first month that it began. That's why I hate to ever work with her again. You may think this doesn't relate to my home health aide story, but sorry it does because had my country not been also dilapidated by them, I won't be here today, tortured by Audrey and her friends.

Even as the U.N. itself and other organizations qualify the displacement of people in Ambazonia as the worst humanitarian crises in recent history, the four year inaction of the media outfits and world bodies charged with policing such happenings has watered down the respect many had for them. Is it because they have something at stake here or just due to the fact that they are glad seeing us all dead so they can come grab our resources? My thoughts are crowded every day with what I see in that country.

I am sick of hearing Audrey and company call me now, minute by minute, just because they know I have been locked indoors for weeks, glued to books, the TV, and my phone, all ears and eyes on any signs or word of hope from President Trump, New York's Mayor Cuomo, or from our governor, who seems to be snoring and saying nothing. But unfortunately all that comes out of their mouths foretells doom, casting thicker clouds over my roof, the streets, and city.

DRASTIC U-TURN

Tall, beautiful skyscrapers that made New York rock 24/7, the *New York Times* edifice, and Time Square with its gigantic flashing billboards announcing the latest movies in the great USA have all gone dead within days. Yet Audrey wants me to drive to such a desolate place, this one-time most powerful booming city on earth turned grave-yard overnight? I never heard this kind of story in history, not even in the Bible. Noah was ready for the flood, and the people were all swept away in a kind of whirlwind flood without being traumatized this way.

Makes me laugh when I hear of all those super-visors who illtreated me most, muster the courage to tell me to go drive through New York City now. I asked her if she didn't hear about the thousands of daily deaths there. If she wasn't aware of the death of 49-year-old Dr. Lorna M. Been, who after treating so many covid patients at the New York-Presbyterian Allen Hospital, rushed home to her parents in Virginia and committed suicide. The director of the emergency room doing that tells how ravaging this pandemic is. Her father said she was such a dedicated medical doctor and had been working twelve to eighteen hours a day since the corona outbreak before her strange action prompted by the heaps of corpses, the sight of which she couldn't stand any longer. She decided to quit the horror by inflicting suicidal wounds on herself. To hell with Audrey's proposed double pay. Nonsense! Now she thinks of giving me $28/hour. Tells how serious this must be.

That cannot buy my life. It's scary out there. Getty of my other agency is also offering me the same pay rate as the director's? That's tempting! This is the very same Audrey to whom I cried for eight years running for a pay raise, and for the first time last month, she added a paltry $0.50 to my $10.50 per hour income. My colleague Colette on $11/hour for thirteen years was granted a derisory $0.85 raise last year.

Thank God she stopped calling me finally. One week gone already! Prrrrrrrrrmmmm. "Sandy, are you ok?"

Reluctantly I shudder, and then answer her call, "Yes."

She sounds desperately beaten up by something. This time, she's actually weeping. "I too caught the virus. Just been nowhere else but to and from the office for the past four weeks to follow up placement of staff."

My heart starts beating like a tantrum dance drum sound. It's bleeding. The company has more than seven hundred home-based customers. All of them depending on the HHAs to come and assist them each day. Audrey is one of the main coordinators in charge of assigning the aides.

"I am in self-quarantine. I had transferred all office equipment needed here, to work from home. Please, are you available now to help me with one of the cases?" she beckons, sobbing in a faint voice.

The question sinks deep through my spine, pushing me into a drastic turnaround without second thought, "Yes, Audrey."

On the edge of her grave and Audrey still is thinking of saving our own frail mothers and fathers? What a sacrifice she has had to make for these elderly people to find herself in this devastating state. My 76-year-old mum is there in Sierra Leone, and I pray every day for COVID not to get close to her.

"Nothing will happen to me as I jump out here to assist her mates," I thought, with the popular phrase "one good turn deserves another" coming to mind. Then knelt down and prayed, "May you, Divine King, open their minds, eyes, and ears to perceive all the ills and maltreatment they have put me and my countrymen and women through in this job. Also give them a turnaround in the evil plans they are cooking against my people, especially those on the African continent, with this white 'fabricated corona monster' as most of our people call it. In my continent, similar accusations rage against them for bringing HIV/AIDS and ebola to exterminate us, but you, Our Most Honored Creator, saved us from their worst. And will continue doing so as there is no power greater than yours in this universe."

After this prayer, I immediately called her with an urgent response, "Audrey, this is Sandy. I am ready to shoot out for the case in New York, and any other critical cases around there, to work as many hours as my body will be able to take. Don't worry about how much to pay me."

FLORA ABANDONED

I am Flora, 91 years old, of Italian nationality. I thank God for preserving my faculties and giving me the energy that permits me to tell you the whole story. I thank Him for the strength He provides me daily to take a shower, make my own food, brush my hair, and do a lot of other things for myself. But then, I have always had a care-giver because I am a fall risk due to a recent knee surgery. Most times, I would reject being sent one until I got stuck and then I understood how important these HHAs are.

I used to be so selective about what kind of aide should be sent to me, but I have humbled myself to Christ's level this time. I wept like a baby to my agency to find me one during the COVID-19 outbreak and felt fire when they couldn't. They told me that most of their aides were refusing to work. I kept calling and they tried hard each day. When nothing was forthcoming, that made me full of anxiety thinking of how I could get rot any time on my bed. Despite that, nursing home or assisted living facilities were still the worst options to me.

I am not afraid of death. But I just dream of dying in a decent way. Having someone nearby to gently help me prepare for it and put myself together at that final hour. That can't be so in some of those nursing homes or assisted living residences that I know, where everything with the aides seems to be in a deafeningly frantic rush without much care for interpersonal relationship with the residents.

I have invested so much in this life not only materially but also spiritually and wouldn't want to miss salvation or a better world after because of a minor last minute mistake that I must have made these horrific days. That's the reason why I need a caregiver in here with me to communicate with on these rising concerns and assist me stay comfortable and calm. None is forthcoming.

I have been all by myself for twenty-one days now. My only daughter is far away in Kentucky. No flights running for her to come take me over. They are all locked up like us for months. Even if there is a flight, would she take it, when for over five years she couldn't pay me a visit? Her job has been more valuable to her than her own parents. When her father passed away last year, I saw her after those five years, and she is just one hour away from me by air.

COVID-19 has been sent by God to pound home the message of how useless all that work, money, and wealth accumulation can suddenly become. See how useless their cars, houses, schools, and companies have become at the twist of a button? Who could ever imagine this in his wildest dreams? First in the history of mankind. If there is anyone out there who doesn't believe what the Bible says about the last days, then let him sit up, for this is a micro glimpse of the end time tsunami. Luke 21:11 of the Christian bible admonishes that, *"There will be great earthquakes, and in various places famines and pestilences. And there will be terrors and great signs from heaven"*. If anyone doubted the might of God, then this is time to rethink. If anyone was ever neglecting what He commands us to do to be true children of His, then this is the time for us to adjust our wicked, greedy ways.

Had those agencies been doing that, then I wouldn't be sitting here nervous all day for three weeks now because no aide is avabilale for me. And they told me many other clients of theirs are in the same nightmare. The caregivers would not be rejecting work as much as they are doing now.

My caregivers have been my husband, my companions, my children, my comforters - in short, the loves of my life.

Thank God that these days I haven't fallen as I often do. What if it so happens? Then these frail bones will all be shattered. I dread that. If my aide Eliza steps in that door today, she will appear to be more than angel to me. It's now I can see how much beauty of heart most of them that I called bitches and poor, and that I lied about for stealing my things and causing them to be fired had. My own child has never given me half the compassion and care that I have received from some of them. Honestly, given what they do for us, they are supposed to be paid more than those sitting behind the desks in the offices, churning papers and assigning these caregivers. See how they run around from home to home, putting smiles on our faces at a time we need them most.

Had they been treated as good as they deserve, then the agencies would not be facing such hard times trying to influence them to go work in the midst of COVID. This teaches us, the clients, to also start appreciating what they do for us. Had we been doing that, then we would have been surprised to find them calling us and the agency to come help us and not the other way round. This should be a big lesson for one to prepare better against any other such horror.

It is thanks to them that the agencies exist. If it's possible for us all to hire the caregivers directly, those agencies wouldn't be alive. Imagine that I pay $350 each day to the agency and they give my aide, who serves me all day, $110/day. How unfair! If I were to hire and pay her directly, she would be having at least twice that amount and I too would have much of that money left in my wallet.

Of course, all clients cannot hire directly, but their employers should treat them better when they get all that money from us. We know they have the cost of paperwork, office staff, and space to cover. But those are not good enough reasons for them to pay the HHAs so low or abusively. Ask why agency A will pay my aide $110/day and agency B pays her $150/day for the same amount of work. I know that because these are two agencies with which I signed contracts for the same HHA service at different times. More so, my friend is having an aide from the other agency right now and giving them exactly what I used to pay there. Yet her aide still receives $110/day.

In case I live after this nightmare, I will never again treat these children the way I used to do. They are true heroes of our society, for there is no better, honorable job to do than that of taking care of your elderly parents who go through thick and thin for you to be where you are today. And more so when you think you will get there one day and expect someone to look after you the same way and with minimal respect, what other blissful thought can you have about these caregivers?

They deserve our honor and respect. See how they go out there in homes of former physicists, doctors, professors, former heads of states, pilots, engineers, astronauts, etc., to take care of them and even control these homes sometimes.

I remember these beautiful African proverbs saying, "Every woman is a mother to all children," and "One person gives birth to a child, but it takes a village to bring him up." So we have to treat them all like our own children without race and color considerations as they render sacrificial services to us. We need those services so badly at this delicate stage of our lives. If we expect decent, fair treatment from them, especially in the face of another corona outbreak, we must be fair too. And most importantly, without trying to produce doubtful vaccines and weapons aimed at destroying or exterminating their people because they are of another breed. So, we can have it all for ourselves." Flora ends her talk in a decision that she will not go back to her agency when things get to normal.

Almost 30,000 deaths in New York alone in two months, with public agencies and private companies fighting for limited supplies of latex gloves and masks in the U.S, explains how terrifying the COVID-19 outbreak was here.

A Reuters report talked of a Texas-based company operating in twenty-six states that had instructed its caregivers to leave the homes of clients who recently traveled from the states with "widespread community transmission" or who had contact with anyone screened for corona virus, regardless of whether that person tested positive or not. What became of those patients is the hanging question.

At treatment centers, those who were not very sick were sent back home because hospitals could barely contain the rising number of corona cases they already had. If many caregivers refused going to work, then that must have had a fatal effect on homebound clients.

The home healthcare companies should, in the future, make budgetary provisions for stock reserves that can supply them with protective gear for months in case of another such pandemic. Clients could also do the same in their homes.

As the companies were condemning lack of protective gear and financial help for better functioning, many of the aides were quitting the job, abandoning clients. This was so disturbing since it made it difficult for tests to be done fast on suspected cases, nursing fears of a quick spread of the infection.

58 out of 75 caregivers in New Jersey that we called to find out if they went to work during the COVID-19 outbreak said they didn't, almost all giving the same reasons for not doing so like Sandy. 98% said their companies never care about them and wouldn't send a word of sympathy to their families, if covid killed them outhere at work. Out of 50 clients that we questioned, 35 said they had no caregivers to assist them and were either taken against their will to a center for seniors or disabled persons or were helped by family members.

TWO

GOOD PLANNING AT THE START THAT SAVES YOU FROM THE WORST

During my research for this work, a good number of Africans and Latinos questioned on their first job when they arrived in the U.S. mentioned home health care. For some, it has been a springboard from which they moved to other trades. Some continue with the job indefinitely or for as long as they live in the country. I met many others who even after going for further studies to obtain big certificates and degrees still keep their home care jobs alongside new ones related to their new professions.

"I am a social worker, but I have decided to preserve my home health care job for the past eight years," said Angela Aden. "It's a job in which you can avoid stress the way you want. Also, I stay on it due to its flexible nature. That's one of the rare professions in this country where you can take time off work when you want, return from vacation when you can, and still get your job. No one imposes a vacation time limit on you or any other strict regulations on your time management."

Good planning of this time and other aspects of the job at the very start is fundamental for an aide who aims at diverse trades and wants to be spared much stress and humiliation during work life.

After your training, before going out to fill in application forms, do your groundwork. Research and get a list of home care companies and other institutions that recruit aides. Let no one tell you to go apply with company A or B and you jump at it without doing background checks on them as they do on you. You can go through these companies online. Read their history and performances. Find out from friends in the industry and those who have been there what they know or have heard people say about them. After doing this search, then you can go about applying. At least you will be picking a company that is more likely to live up to your expectations.

There are hundreds of others out there with doors ready to welcome you into the world of mistreatment. Don't fall into their hands thoughtlessly. If you do that at the onset and they begin to disappoint you, when you leave them it's like you carry a curse along that places barriers on your way to any other company that may treat you better.

"I know many colleagues who have experienced that as they move from agency to agency in New Jersey," Larissa who is HHA since three years confirmed. "Some of them divorcing with five to ten agencies in a year because of ill-treatment from the recruiter or the client."

Another good item to compare at the beginning is pay rates of the different agencies so you can choose the best for yourself. The pay ranges from

$10/hour to $18/hour for companies or clients who hire privately.

Some private clients will even pay more than that. While in the field working, you will always come across employees who have private clients. If not, look out for them during your interpersonal relationships. Discuss the topic with them and they will open up to give insight into these private cases. If you are not the kind of person with a friendly disposition who can make co-workers feel comfortable near you to welcome a conversation, then forget it; just coil up in your shell and remain miserable during your lifetime on that job. But if you are a little outgoing, carrying a smile along, you will be able to find colleagues who can open up to you and help you learn much, letting you know what to do in order to find something better.

"When colleagues notice you are full of yourself, that makes them hide many things from you," Larissa warned. "It's a profession in which we must always hold each other's hand, to be able to stand those uphill challenges encountered with the many ungrateful employers and their clients. Many of them enjoy threatening, firing us, and firing at us." At some point, that may become traumatizing to aides who are ignorant of their rights like some newbies. You need to have an iron spine to be able to stand the trials at times.

Even if a company is proposing double what another company is offering, do not rush to that and neglect the other. Aides recount how some of these companies that pay relatively higher are hardly consistent in giving you work. They will offer you a case today, and when you lose it, they tell you to be patient and wait for a call when something else is available. There you go hoping, but when you start waiting, it can take weeks or months. You are tempted to patiently wait because within that period they could occasionally call to propose cases that you cannot do because of distance or other reasons.

"I have the impression that most do that deliberately, to discourage you from your repeated calls to remind about your wait," said Andrew, an aide. That is true. It's a trick by some of them just to satisfy you when you call persistently. Some will propose a case that doesn't fulfill the conditions that you indicated you wanted during your hiring interview.

Therefore, avoid falling for the big pay and neglecting the lesser pay without extensive analyses and proper inquiry. Those offering average pay can be more consistent in giving you cases when you lose a client. At times, you don't go for one or two weeks before being offered another case.

"I used to wonder how my agency always succeeded," Andrew observed. "We are over 2,000 employees in the company, but you cannot lose a job and go for two weeks without them calling you back to work. I was with them for seven years without losing work for ten days at any given moment."

CLIENT

If you are in the process of subjecting yourself to the services of a home health agency or aide, you too need elaborate planning months ahead of time. This will greatly reduce your stress with upcoming complications in your rapport with them and the many people and institutions that you will be dealing with. Without doing so, You will wrack your brains almost every day.

Once you make a good plan even years before, you can be sure that peace, tranquility, and happiness shall accompany you.

The first thing to do is to put yourself together mentally, emotionally, psychologically, and physically. You are going to be meeting different types of people. You will be working with them day after day as they become almost part of your family. Your relatives may be far away and you not seeing them often, but the home health aides are there to fill that vacuum. So be ready to embrace them with love and positive energy. If not, you will find yourself in misery and sometimes absolute doom that could gradually become fatal if that rejection or racist spirit keeps clouding your thoughts.

Before inviting the services of the caregiver, do your complete health check. If you have any transmissible diseases, take effective treatment ahead of the aide's arrival. Let your conscience lead you into doing that. Don't expect someone to come tell you to do it; don't expect your agency to tell you to do it; don't wait for the aide to get infected and fall sick before you start taking precautions for the next aide.

"I'm bed bound for four years because of a chronic disease that I contracted from one of our clients," said Nora, working as caregiver for eignt years.

"Neither the agency nor I knew she had it. She hid that from us because she must have feared being denied service. It was while in bed that I called my colleagues to tell them that I was sick, and they informed me they too at some time had suffered from the same illness that I had, and the agency dismissed them so they shouldn't infect the client. Ironically!"

From Nora's account, she was the third to be infected by the client, and it was much later when her client was diagnosed with the same disease that she could trace the source of her illness.

She had been in a very cordial relationship with the client's relations, and they maintained ties when she got bedridden and were visiting her with gifts time and again. They were surprised to learn from her that during four years of her being home, her company had called just once to know if she was available for work and never called again to find out about the progress of her health, despite having knowledge of the critical illness eating her up.

This brings up the question from most aides on why clients are not forced to do thorough medical exams like the caregivers are obliged to do. Aren't they supposed to be doing that for the safety of these caregivers?

If the agency cared just a little about Nora and her colleagues and had concern for their health as much as they did for their clients, then from the first infected case, they could have discovered more about this to be able to stop the spread and avoid the worst for these aides. Who knows if some of the infected ones ended up dying.

YOUR FILES AND BILLS

Also put together all files that will have something to do with your caregiving and day-to-day running of your life activities - medical files, cable bills, telephone bills, bank transactions, house ownership documents, mortgage files, power of attorney documents, insurance files, etc. Arrange them very well and classify them distinctly in a safe drawer. If you can't because of frailty or failing health, invite an expert bookkeeper to do the job. Once this is done, you won't imagine how much good sleep you will have going to bed every day, confident that all your records are straight. That way, in the days that follow, whenever an issue crops up relating to any of these files, it's easy for you to pick up what you need.

Many in your state have been victims of exorbitant or fabricated bills that they cannot explain because they are unable to think well and trace where the receipts and documents scattered in different spots of the house are. Sometimes getting these papers together sends them into total confusion. Because of that, you find some clients in stage one dementia degenerate to stage three in less than no time. People who stop by are amazed and ask what suddenly happened to her - question that usually only the aide of the client can answer.

Have a diet calendar outlining your feeding time-table, especially the foods you often prefer. This calendar can cover a month, meaning the schedule is repeated at the end of each month. That way the aide doesn't have to ask questions each time you request something to eat when you are unable to prepare food for yourself.

You will need to do the same with your medications. As you get older in Western countries, prepare your mind psychologically for heavy pill consumption if you are ignorant of home reme-dies. No one in your chain of medical care will want to listen as they struggle to impose medica-tions that you might not have need for. Victims say that is done because it is their cash cow for wealth building and not absolutely because of a disturbing ailment that requires you taking these medications. You escape their trap only if you are a strong-willed person to refuse them imposing on you. If you aren't one, then get ready for the volumes of meds or, at the least, for nutritional supplements.

"What they keep insisting you take makes you feel that's your life wire and you are tempted to accept," Emelda, an 80-year-old mother complained. "Look at this tray of med boxes. Full of capsules and tablets that I drink Monday to Sunday, morning. afternoon, evening, night. And at least seven pills at each swallowing session since five years. What's the meaning of all these?" Many of her peers have often asked this question.

Why only in America and most of the Western nations do we find that? Go to other countries, especially in Africa or parts of Asia and you won't see this happening. Its easy there to find an old mother with all her teeth gone at age 100 without a single pill or nutritional supplement on her bedside table, without having been on any pills in the last twenty years. Yet she will be ok with just minor age-related ailments.

"What is all this pill consumption for, with the torture some of us go through as we absorb those packs of tablets and capsules each blessed day," said Grandma Hannah, jittery. "Makes you have no taste for food or life at times, just thinking your life is kind of hanging on a scale, to collapse the minute you stop swallowing pills. The psychological torture from that is excessive."

Some of this torture is inflicted just to satisfy the predatory quest of a pharmaceutical witch hunter somewhere in high quarters and not because the patients really need the pills.

This is why friends or family members have to often come in to save the elderly from their claws when they are getting too vulnerable and cannot make certain crucial decisions by themselves. Come in to study what is going on and save them from the claws of any moguls. Do an analysis of whatever the nurses, doctors, physical therapists, and the rest are proposing to them before accepting that your relation (the client) gets drowned into it.

Another set of exploiters are some physical therapists who will recommend exercises that you don't need in order to come around for a long period of time to assist you with a few stretches and go loaded. Some will keep lying that you need more sessions for healing from an accident that caused you a light, harmless fracture. They will extend physical therapy that was supposed to last weeks to several months on these fragile people, just for the sake of God knows what.

CLEANLINESS, NEXT TO GODLINESS

Another thing you have to get ready for as you prepare to welcome the services of a home health aide is engaging in thorough cleaning of all the nooks and crannies of your home. If you are not strong enough to do that, get the services of a cleaning agency or agent. And continue requesting their services frequently or occasionally.

An unclean house full of litter will make you sicker than before, especially when you have to spend more of your time in there than outside. Most of us know how comfortably we sleep like a baby each night that we change our bed sheets and look around to see the room and house impeccably neat. You must do everything to avoid hoarding. It's sickening to see things hanging all over your head.

A stuffy, unclean house will make your home health aide also sick and uncomfortable. And some whom you would like so much to stay with you may decide to take an impromptu leave with a lame excuse and never come back no matter how hard you try. You can keep losing good services of great aides because of the outlook of your house.

Some clients insist on nothing being moved from the hoarded mess even if it stands in the way of effective service of the aide and others who come in to help or visit.

The service chart of almost all agencies clearly states that apart from activities of daily living and personal care to offer the client, a caregiver has to do only very light cleaning of essential spaces used by both. And light cleaning means keeping clean all used items/areas (including bathroom, kitchen and the areas where the client sits and sleeps) before the aide returns home.

The client has the responsibility for general cleaning of her residence and care of her pets and garden, which should be a must in order to guarantee the health of both parties.

THREE

ABUSES AND CLIENTS TURNING YOU INTO A SHOCK ABSORBER

You meet clients of all ages, shades, colors, and bizarre temperaments in the field. Even though home health care is generally thought to be centered on the elderly, younger people with pertinent health issues that need long-lasting solutions and others get assistance too. Children with physical or mental defects are also clients.

When going out to serve them, be ready for the good, the bad, and the ugly. If you are not psychologically prepared for these, then start metamorphosing into a shock absorber. If you can't, you may never make it. All kinds of cases await you at strange places. If you aren't employed in a facility, more often than not, you are not seated on a spot to work but out in the field shuttling from one home to the next. Whenever you arrive at a client's residence, be ready for the worst and let the good come to you as a surprise. This way, little or nothing shocks or dissuades you from any case to which you are assigned.

"Many of the elderly clients that I met are some of the nicest people you can think of," caregiver Clara affirmed. "But when you handle them abusively, don't be surprised to see them give you the ugliest treatment imaginable."

During their good mood, most are welcoming, warm, and conversational, with a lot of entertaining and educational stories to share with you. Their experiences will enrich and teach you how to go about the rising mishaps of this sick world, how better to manage your profession, your marriage, your children and family.

They have a wealth of knowledge that you can never get from a classroom, given to you freely. That is the reason why as we grow up, we need to always go looking for them, not expecting them to call us before we create time to visit them.

Here you will learn how aides manage some of these surprises and shocks.

THE AMPUTATED GRANDMOTHER

(as narrated by Clara)

This amputee was one of my very first cases when I started the profession. It was with a company all the way in Ocean City, NJ. No one had explained the kind of case awaiting me.

I was hurriedly assigned by the office, and being in dire need of a job, I jumped for it. Not driving then, someone rushed to take me there. That day we meandered through a country road for over two hours to arrive a retreated green glowing Jewish community with an eerie quiet that got me tongue tight for hours. I was dropped off to stay for three months without going back home. Fright enveloped my thoughts as I stepped out of the car to the whistling breeze and mass tweets of birds lining very tall trees, no human in sight. The many twists and bends of the trajectory had kept my heart pounding all along. That was the first time that I'm taken to this kind of assignment called live-in since I arrived this country months ago.

"'What if he is taking me to dump off where no one will ever see me again? What if he stops somewhere and rapes me? What if he kills me on the way?' These questions were haunting me all along with no one to answer or give me assurance of my safety as I have almost no acquaintance in the U.S. Even when I took off at the agency, no one gave me this assurance.

The first day I arrived, 79-year-old Mrs. Esther was welcoming. We had a brief good conversation while she was lying in bed. It wasn't until I had to start assisting her to move that I realized her two legs were amputated. It was so embarrassing because no one had hinted [at it to] me. There wasn't much I could do at that point because the person who accompanied me was already gone. And being a weekend, I couldn't reach the office by phone easily. Even if I did, how could I start complaining after staying home for so long without a job? I thought I could just continue and struggle to do the work.

You can imagine how hard it was for an inexperienced home health aide like me at her very first task. I was supposed to help her up with her crutches but didn't just know how to do it, having never had any training on this. She didn't want to understand any explanations or make any effort to understand my professional handicap as I struggled to do with her physical handicap. The frustration and bitterness that brewed up in us couldn't be contained for long before bursting out, leading to my departure.

KEEPING KOSHER

Eleanor's own surprise in another Jewish home was food related. According to the law, feeding of home health aides on live-in assignments should be taken care of by the client. She narrated how "they insisted that as Orthodox Jews, I needed to absolutely respect the kosher law like them. I wanted to leave that same day of my arrival, but the office begged me hard as they had no one for replacement.

It's true we have to be culturally tolerant in this profession but not in extreme cases like this one. How could they force me, a fervent born-again Christian, to so suddenly start abiding 100 percent to their kosher laws when under their roof? What a cultural shock, given the unbecoming impression that I had about the Jewish while growing up! Eating nothing but their kosher foods, when I had all these Kwene village delicacies that I had brought, stuck up in my bags?"

The kitchen was a no-go zone, with strict rules of what to cook on which stove and what to wash in what sink. To note that these were apportioned to the kitchen sections with dairy products and the section with meat products. She wasn't even allowed to cook any of her delights, touch a stove, or wash her own dish because she could Violate a kosher law.

After three weeks of starvation there, Eleanor returned home lost seven pounds.

THERAPY FROM GRACE'S SPIRIT AND SMILES

(as narrated by her aide Thelma)

Grace was the most cheerful ninety-something-year-old I ever came across. For the one month that I spent with her, not even once did I see her face dark or red. She would yell at you to do something for her but in a cheerful manner. She always appeared lucid and you could see in her someone who had been happy all her life. On reaching her home at 2 p.m. from two very difficult clients that I cater for in the mornings, Grace always deleted the scars of their torments from my face before I reached home to my family.

She told me she never had a child or husband. When I asked of her secret in healing my wounds, she responded, 'Because I always do to others what I would want them do to me, often smiled, always thank my creator for everything about my life; hardly regret why I don't have this or that; ate a clean, balanced diet throughout, never went into excesses and always showed love. That primarily, is what makes you a complete human being and success story. Not the cars, jets, houses or degrees that you possess."

She wouldn't let you do what she could try to do for herself, even if it would take her one hour to do what you would do in five minutes. She is 90 plus years old, but independence to her is the golden word. She hates seeing you try to take control of her movements even as she uses a walker. Her faculty is as fresh as that of a woman decades younger. The fact that I told her my name just once, and for the two years that I spent with her, she never asked me to remind her of it, tells you all.

Grace recounted her life story eloquently from her teenage years to date, with vivid description of events. The way she spoke and pulled herself around was revealing of one who had lived a decent, balanced life. She possessed almost all the nine gifts of the Spirit, characteristics of a complete born-again Christian, but had never been to a church. I would wonder if it's because she was blessed with the name Grace.

She wasn't naughty like some grannies but knew her full rights as client. She would request you do something for her only within the precincts of the work schedule assigned to you by your agency.

Mutual respect bred such harmony and love between us that the day I was leaving her, both of us wept in each other's arms. I left after two years just because I had to go to school."

AWKWARD BATHS

Gloria, a 28 year old caregiver snapped, "It was so embarrassing when I found myself before this huge 6.5-foot-tall Mr. Kingsley, in his late seventies, giving him a sponge bath. He had hair all over his body, and it was like you tickled him each time you touched a grain of that hair. He would go yelling as I gave his bath, with a coarse voice that broke through the roof." But she often than not maintained some patience.

"Whenever I slid the sponge down the penis area to clean, he would jump and give the loudest scream, sometimes even giggling. Anyone out of the house could think I was doing something wrong to him. It was usually so embarrassing and got me worried all along because neighbors were listening, and I feared there could be misinterpretations even if they signaled the police and I explained." She needed a big heart to stand it all.

"The situation was even worse and more disturbing each time I found myself pulling the tip of his penis out as he sat on the chair, to fit into the urinal for him to pee. You won't imagine he would pee about fifteen times in the day, and as for the night, I shouldn't start narrating. It was just hell."

JACKY'S COSTLY ABUSE

There is this pathetic story of an 82-year-old that I came across who had entrusted everything including her financial records, debit and credit cards in the hands of her aide, Jacky because she was in charge of her shopping.

When this young girl of twenty-nine years started using the bank cards of the lady for her personal shopping without the client's knowledge, no one around her was aware. She used it to pay her bills and gas at pump stations for months.

Bills were coming to the elderly lady's address, and she was paying them. At some point, the expenses rose so high that she called for a third party to check out the books with her. They were shocked to realize that for eight months this young girl was using the client's cards for her personal purchases. They discovered bills related to consumption of electricity, water, gas plus more.

The company that had sent her there was also in utter disbelief because they had not done background check on this girl during hiring before she was assigned to the lady with whom she worked for three years. Upon investigation, they found that she had committed a series of felonies that were supposed to disqualify her for the job. She was arrested, her license revoked, and was charged heavy penalties. How jeopardizing that was to her career and future search for a new job cannot be overemphasized. It's a big lesson to others who are going down her route or who join the profession with plans to exploit.

It is at your own risk and peril as an aide to try duping an elderly father or mother because, come what may, one day you will be caught red-handed, which could land you into dismal misery for a long time. And you may never recover from such an act in a country like the U.S. where your activities are all bundled in a transparent glass building.

FOUR

REVERSING SOUR EXPERIENCES

These caregivers can reverse the tides by also planting their financial tentacles in business arenas of their communities, to also offer jobs that will bring back their money turning in their own hands. That can eventually change their story as their lives turn around.

Ownership of the home health-care companies in most states in the U.S. seems to be a thing of some privileged class or race that doesn't do up to 5 percent of the delicate jobs that this industry offers. Out of the 280 aides interviewed for this book, only 7 percent were of the white race. And only 10 percent of their clients were black folks. The aides were sampled in the tri-state areas of New York, New Jersey and Pennsylvania, The caregivers were met in home settings where they work, assisted living facilities, day care and seniors' centers. The aides were picked from these places.

If Nana, a caregiver from Ghana, could start her own company, you too can. She worked with the home health-care industry in New Jersey where she had nothing like a promotion or reasonable pay increase for ten years. "I ran around the place to help our clients in the same clothes for one year because I had the burning desire for my freedom from them. I had to drop all other material priorities."

Nana had worked so hard for her boss, the company owner, earning his trust like no other co-worker did. He could count on her for any odd hour of work or emergencies. But despite that, he never thought of improving her status financially and otherwise. She would ask him what it takes to establish such a company and get it to succeed, but he always brushed her question off. As she kept insisting, he told her to stop dreaming because she could never create one.

"I couldn't stand it anymore, doing all those energy-absorbing tasks and long hours, hardly having sleep, sometimes twenty-four hours to cover, only to have a peanut $11/hour wage." the twenty-four hour shift is usually live-in, which doesn't allow sleeping when the client has to when the client has to wake up frequently at night for one thing or another, and you have to watch over him or her.

State regulations stipulate that caregivers can work until bedtime for the client, then go to sleep till the next day. But this can't be possible when you have a client with fall risk or other complications who constantly gets up at night. "Many of my colleagues go through this, but when some of the companies pay you their stipulated $110 per day for live-in, they hardly ever look into all of that."

Nana was so smart that she refused to stay on and continue pinching her fingers for months after months like some aides do while accepting such pay or less for years without even an annual wage increase.

"Yes, some of them are treated like objects," Mike, an elderly client, confirmed. "I have been with these agencies for almost twenty years and know what I am talking about. I constantly discuss with the caregivers and hear their stories. All my life, I had worked so hard and made several investments. Having no wife and children, I signed this contract with the company to which I pay $450/day for their services. But they have never paid any of my aides more than $120/day. It's also annoying and depressing, seeing how you are spending this much on home healthcare, yet the state that is supposed to protect you sometimes applies multiple methods of thievery to grab all your life earnings when you have no one as heir, just like me."

The stingy pay sounded more than ridiculous to Nana, which is the reason why she banged the door to go out and make a difference. And her company is exemplifying that difference in the home health industry, with her $13.50/hour start pay rate for workers.

STICKING NECK FROM THE CROWD

One day, she met her former boss at a New Jersey state meeting of all owners of home health-care companies in the state. Well-clad in a classy professional outfit, she walked up to him and stretched out a hand in greeting. "Hello sir, how are you doing?"

"Hi. Who're you?"

"You don't recognize me? I'm Nana, now owner of a company like yours; that's why am here."

"Whaaat!" She said you could see the shock all over his face.

Nana is now talked of and treated with much respect by her former boss, her partners in the industry, her workers, and clients. She who started just some three years ago commands more respect than many who have been there for decades not only because of her achievements, but also due to the humane treatment she reserves for her workers and clients. An example is her wage pay of between $13.50 and $16 an hour, unlike other companies that have been there for twenty years and still pay around $10 - $12 an hour with an abusive wage increase of $2 for aides who are with them for the same number of years. Meanwhile, they are making millions of dollars yearly off the sweat of these caregivers.

Nana is always all hands on the job. Where the aide has limitations, she drops everything and rushes off to the field to assist him or her. That is why her clients love her much. They are confident of being in safe hands when they sign a contract with Nana's agency.

She takes enough time off to drill them on the highs and lows they should be expecting as they start the ride into home health care.

"Before my aide came, I was already prepared psychologically, morally, physically, and financially to take the challenges one day at a time," said Susan, one of her clients. The immune boosting effect of such preparation cannot be underestimated. "Without that, I could have been overwhelmed to death by these challenges, which seem to multiply daily. I mean very early death."

Nana doesn't change aides of clients as often as many others do, but she concentrates her time more in seeking ways of offering optimum, satisfactory services, good pay, plus incentives.

DISRESPECT OF RULES

The aide may have time flexibility but little flexibility with set rules for the work to which he or she is assigned. Even if the home health agencies don't respect application of some rules in hiding, they try hard not to let observers, the client, and her family members notice this. They would preach to the caregivers, clients, and partners on how ethical values in home health services must not be violated, but many of these agencies are the first to violate them. They would emphasize that the delicate nature of most of their clients requires no one fools around with the strict rules.

The intense pressure on you to respect these rules from your office coordinators and clients could be appreciated but are sickening at times when they overstretch abusively. The office tells you for example not to make phone calls at work. During a 12 hour shift the client watches closely to be sure you respect that. If for a minute you pick up an emergency call, some start yelling. The next day you may hear your boss telling you to quit the case because she had reported that you spent all the time on the phone. Some agencies tell you not to even cover your eyes during a night shift while the client is comfortably sleeping all night. First thing on stepping into a client's home is to wash your hands, which is good for the safety of both parties. No touching of her private items without her permission and many other restrictions. You have clients who will sing these rules into your ears until you can take it no more and are forced to resign.

When you do, most companies find more blame with you than with the client, even when they know she is wrong. You can go and lick your wound; that's not their business. They will find another aide for her as soon as possible in order not to lose the case. Even if they have to offer caregivers to a client who is specialized in rejecting seven different aides in seven days, some agencies keep pushing more to them instead of trying to stop their misconduct by bringing them to reason.

FIVE

TRAINING AND RECRUITMENT

Training to become a home health aide takes place in a school or within the home care company that wants to hire you. It lasts between three and eight weeks, depending on the curriculum design of the trainer and the cost of training. The fee usually ranges from US$300 to US$600.

The course outline covers, amongst other subjects, grooming, assisting clients to bathe, the Health Insurance Portability and Accountability Act (HIPAA), and precautions against infectious diseases, which falls under the Occupational Safety and Health Act (OSHA). It establishes a system of laws to promote and regulate workplace safety.

The training goes with a lot of practicals, and at the end of it, you gather much knowledge on how to manage not only the client's personal care, but yours as well. It gives education on many life-related care needs that we often take for granted.

During recruitment, you do an orientation test with a series of at least 150 questions in all the areas that your training touched. The long hours spent at orientation and interviews illustrate how rigorous assessment for hiring can be in most places.

Over 80% of companies that you contact for recruitment get you through a two- to three-hour test. They apply this rigor in order to avoid the unexpected happening to their client who will be under your care, many of whom can be very delicate. This is followed by a number of medical tests like those for tuberculosis, mumps, rubella; a physical exam; and, most often, a drug test. This test is very important and needs to always be required because a caregiver with a history of drug abuse could be a potential danger to the clients.

Recruits meet a majority of these clients in home settings and stay all day or for very long hours with them depending on the nature of the case, assisting in activities of daily living like showering, cooking, grooming, reminding them of medications to take, and more.

Be it in a two-room apartment or a ten-room mansion, you may often find just two people there, the caregiver and the client. And they could be there for months without anyone stopping by. That is why taking ample precaution to be sure the aide can be trustworthy is quite important. The client may be in that partnership for an undetermined period of time with the caregiver, who may have access to the lifetime assets of the client. That is why trust is absolutely necessary. Some go for as long as ten to fifteen years together.   .

SIX

DEMENTIA AND ALZHEIMER'S CASES: UNDERSTAND THEM WELL BEFORE ENGAGING

The home health aides are called to the field to cater to all sorts of clients - tall, short, sick, well, blind, the deaf, autistic, physically and mentally disabled, and especially those with dementia, Alzheimer's, Parkinson's, or Huntington's disease. Some of the illnesses are so complex that you need to be well schooled to understand how a client is grappling with the disease before engaging in the case. Disregarding this might end up getting you wrecked in a worse state of depression or health complications than the sick client.

Alzheimer's is a chronic, irreversible brain disorder that progresses slowly. It is a neurodegenerative disease that destroys memory, thinking skills, and reasoning, and it worsens over time. The loss of connections between nerve cells in the brain results in messages that are unable to be transferred between these nerve cells in the brain and from the brain to muscles and organs in the body.

According to a Zubican research, symptoms of Alzheimer's disease will usually appear during our mid-sixties. It is estimated that about 5.7 million Americans were living with Alzheimer's disease in 2018. The disease causes 60-70 percent of cases of dementia. Alzheimer's disease is one of the top six causes of death in the United States. (1)

The research states that having a family member develop Alzheimer's is one of the most difficult situations a family can be put in. It's such a painful disease because it will seem like nothing is amiss and then suddenly it will look like your family member is a completely different person.

This back and forth becomes very difficult and painful to see.

Research continues every day around the world to attempt to battle Alzheimer's and alleviate the suffering of the people who have it. Alzheimer's often requires a lot of assistance.

DEMENTIA VS. ALZHEIMER'S

Neither dementia nor Alzheimer's have any treatment. Still, according to the Zubican research, a lot of people confuse dementia with Alzheimer's disease. It can be complicated and things can be mixed up quite easily. Dementia is the umbrella term. Alzheimer's is a common cause of dementia. Think of it this way. If someone is diagnosed with a fever, that would be equivalent to a dementia diagnosis. However, the cause of the fever isn't immediately known. It could be caused by one of many different things. A cause of dementia is Alzheimer's disease.

Memory loss is the first major sign of Alzheimer's, followed by difficulty in performing daily activities, lack of interest in things that used to matter to you, and change in physical abilities amongst others. 54% of the 280 caregivers interviewed for this work said their clients had Alzheimer's or dementia and 37% complained of not having been informed about the state of their client before being sent to them.

Majority of the aides interviewed for this work, who were assigned to dementia or memory loss cases said on setting out to work, some agencies show concern, to think of giving you a detailed report on the new client you are to meet. Others don't care. For them, things just have to go fast so they can catch the money. Even if the client has critical dementia that can get you into danger, whether she weighs 400 pounds and you are just 100 pounds, they don't care, as they ask you to go try to lift her up. All that matters is your presence at that home to help them cash a $500/day check from her insurance and give you a $100 pittance.

Many aides, especially the new recruits, keep falling prey to this, and when they are hooked or faint as a consequence, no one in the agency is there anymore to sympathize with them or hold their hand to rise.

Here is one of many similar scenarios: Your home health agency calls you up and rushes you to a demented client. She weighs 300 pounds and you weigh just 120 pounds. This client is bed bound and needs lifting for all care you have to give her. No one informs you ahead of time of what awaits you. The aide on duty charged to describe the client's condition to you as you arrive is in a rush to leave and doesn't get into the nitty gritties. She may also avoid telling you the details because she had not been assigned to the case for long and because she feared complaining or refusing the case. That way she will avoid being begrudged by the supervisor and blocked from further assignments. While trying to lift the client up, you injure your spinal cord because she is too heavy for you and is fighting with you at the same time due to her demented state. That becomes solely your business to fix, not that of the company. That is because many of the agencies play a lot of gymnastics in order not to get involved in any workman's compensation for their caregivers.

All expenditures for treatment are to be incurred by the caregiver, most of whom are never given work insurance and cannot afford it from their pockets as a result of low pay. Sometimes the injury can even get you handicapped for life. That will never bother your company to come to your aid. The best you will get when you inform them will be a broad smile with "Oooh sorry. Take good care of yourself," and then a warm goodbye. Ask for even $100 assistance from the agency, that falls on deaf ears. You go home and start licking your wounds all alone, may be for years. Don't expect to hear any of them in that office call to find out how you are doing.

That is why when you are contacted for a case, you should hesitate to land yourself there because you absolutely need a job. Take your time to ask all the questions and get all that you have the right to know about the client. Obtain answers that give you a guarantee to render effective service without risk, service that will be good for the client, for you, and for the company—a three-way win.

1. How old is the client?
2. What is her weight?
3. What is her language and religion?
4. What is her nationality?
5. Is she suffering from any disease? If so, which? Most importantly, does she have dementia ?
6. Is she a fall risk?
7. Does she harbor pets?

8. Is she bedridden?

9. Is she handicapped?

10. Does she like conversation or not?

Here are some of the main questions that, if answered, will clarify you on what you will get. It's not fair for you to discover these answers only when you arrive at the client's home. It is often so embarrassing to both of you when you reach there completely blank on what awaits you. That makes some aides jittery and the client upset, pushing both to start calling the office and complaining about each other. Caregivers who don't have the courage to tell their employer that they cannot continue with the case stay on with anger that breeds conflict with the client as time goes on. When this becomes incurable, replacement, dismissal, sanctions, or sudden abandonment of the case by the caregiver follow. At times, this is done in an abrupt way that can drastically affect the health of the client.

ABRUPT STOPS AFFECT ALL PARTIES

The abrupt stop sometimes gives the agency staff serious headaches to find an appropriate replacement, which may arrive at a time when a client with delicate health and degenerating dementia must have suffered emotional, mental, or psychological shock that raises her blood pressure to stroke level.

Mark stressed, "That's what happened to my 74-year-old mother after deadly arguments with an aide, which cost her life. Not only did her blood pressure rise after that, but she also plunged into a stroke that got her bedridden for the rest of her four last years on this planet." What a disaster! This has happened to so many who could have been spared if precaution was taken.

If the questions above are always properly answered, then half the problems are solved and the agency will go a long way to avoid changing caregivers on one client frequently.

Like Judith Nwaro a 60 year old caregiver recounted, "I went to this client who told me she had had fourteen aides in eight months. Isn't that terrible! How can they leave that happen? It could be quite confusing and depressing to her, the care-givers, and even some of their fragile supervisors who go through the hassle of finding the new aides. She said she is the one who sent away all of them or asked for the changes because their services were below her expectations." And unfortunately, her reasons pointed to almost all the ten questions above.

Susan Barley, coordinator in one of the agencies, said many clients are more complex than we can imagine, and that's why they are forced to accept their wish for changes.

She said, "Even after you provide an aide with answers to all the ten questions, you will find those who will still create complications for her. Some of the clients are by nature troublemakers while others do so because of degenerative memory caused by ailments like dementia, Alzheimer's, or Huntington's disease."

Whatever it may be, it would be wise for you, the aide, to assess the situation in detail and judge if you can stand the whims, caprices, and sometimes outright verbal or physical brutality of the client. If you can't, quit the job. If you don't, that could gradually stress you out to a point where you develop a worse health complication, like what happened to Laura who for 10 years as HHA, did the job with admirable passion and compassion, refusing to get into any other profession.

"I didn't want to be jumping from place to place, hoping with time she would change, given that she had no dementia or Alzheimer's," she said. "The agency had assigned me to seven clients within a month, and I was getting sick about it. I needed some stability. But the abuses from this client were eating me up bit by bit, and I would return home every day like a mad person, kicking at everything as I arrived, including my own child; can you imagine that? The emotional and psychological damage gradually increased and became irreparable."

ENDNOTES
Six

1. *https://www.zubican.com/diseases--conditions/ what-are-the-signs-of-alzheimers*

SEVEN

AS OBTAINED ELSEWERE

When you See how many western families have
lost great values in grandparent care, you feel sorry
for their elderly and even future generations. You
are tempted to tell some of them to travel to Africa
or other continents and learn about some of those
values that keep energizing family bonding there.

In Africa, for example, the grandparent is an
embodiment of wisdom, blessings, compassion,
love, and more. When an elder places his hand on
you and blesses you, you are sure the road ahead
will be open wide for success in your adventures as
you grow up.

The children often find time to go sit near their
grandparent to listen to stories of their lives and
of the evolution of society before they were born.
Relating their life experiences to them helps inspire
and motivate these young ones to step into the

footsteps of the elderly. They find it a wonderful privilege to join conversations with them. And they would also derive much pleasure from assisting them with any activity of daily living, materially and financially, expecting no pay. Or expecting just their blessings as reward.

Most African children who sound smart, intelligent, and wise are those who have had some grooming from grannies. That is why some parents always invite their own parents to come take care of their children or send them to live with the grandparents for upbringing or grooming, if not for always, at least during vacations.

It is often with absolute delight that these grandparents care for the children. And the bond between both parties is usually strong and full of love that is rejuvenating for the granny and emotionally stabilizing for the child. The joy of doing it stimulates the immunity of the grandparents without them being aware, thus lengthening their lives. The love bond eats deep into the psyche of the children, that is why when they grow up, they hardly forget their own parents. They think it a duty to pay back and would hardly neglect their parents or grandparents. It is an interesting, fascinating cycle that makes it difficult for these African children to grow up neglecting their aging parents like many in western countries doing. A similar experience is obtained in other societies as we will find out in Appendix 1 of this book.

APPENDIX I

Stories Of 100+ -Year-Old People: Healthy, Strong, Active, And Working

The captivating findings about these individuals living healthy, strong, and physically active beyond 100 years are presented here in the words of Dan Buettner as he did in a video.

Only about 10 percent of how long the average person lives is dictated by our genes. The other 90 percent is dictated by our lifestyle. The average human body is capable of living for about ninety years. In America, we are leaving about twelve good years on the table.

Scientist found five "blue zones" on earth where people live up to ninety years and beyond: The Seventh Day Adventist Community in Loma Linda, California; Okinawa in Japan; Sardinia in

Italy; Nicoya in Costa Rica; and Ikaria in Greece. There are nine solid reasons for their long lives.

1. THEY DON'T EXERCISE

They don't exercise the way we think of exercising, but they set up their lives in a way that they are constantly nudged into physical activities.

Sardinians live in vertical houses and are up and down the stairs. They don't have any conveniences. There is not a button to push to do yard or house-work. They mix cake by hand, and the people live 100 years with extraordinary vigor. They have places where 102-year-olds still ride their bikes to work, chop wood, and can beat a guy sixty years younger.

2. THEY HAVE A PURPOSE

They have vocabulary for "sense of purpose." In Okinawan language, there is no word for "retirement." Instead there is one word that imbued your entire life and the word is "ikigai," meaning "the reason for which you wake up in the morning." For a 100-year-old fisherman that I talked to, it was continuing to catch fish for his family three times a week. And for a 102-year-old elderly mother, her ikagai is to feed her great-great-great-granddaughter. When I asked how she feels about it, she said it feels like leaping into heaven.

3. THEY RELAX

Each of the five cultures takes time to downshift.

- The Sardinians pray.

- The Seven Day Adventists pray.

- The Okinawans have ancestral veneration.

When you are in a hurry or stressed out, that triggers something called the inflammatory response, which is associated with everything from Alzheimer's to cardiovascular disease.

4. THEY EAT LESS

The greatest diet ever invented is known as the "hara hachu bun me" diet. It's simply a little saying the Okinawans say before their meals that reminds them to stop eating when the stomach is 80 percent full. That's because it takes twenty minutes for the "full feeling" to travel to our brain. And they have all kinds of little strategies to keep them from over eating. They eat off of smaller plates, so they tend to eat fewer calories at every sitting.

5. THEY EAT A PLANT-BASED DIET

Their diets are full of vegetables with lots of color in them. They eat about eight times as much tofu as Americans do. Experts say tofu contains all nine essential amino acids and is a great source of iron. This means they don't eat meat but lots of beans and nuts.

6. THEY FOCUS ON FAMILY

The foundation of all these is how they connect. They put their families first and take care of their children and their aging parents.

Seventh Day Adventists schedule twenty-four hours a week with their loved ones and God. And then hardwired right in their religion are nature walks.

7. THEY HAVE STRONG RELATIONSHIPS

They also belong to the right tribe. They were either born into or they proactively surrounded themselves with the right people.

8. THEY PRAY

They all tend to belong to a faith-based community. Numerous studies have found a link between praying regularly and living longer. One study found that attending services regularly can add an average of four years to a person's life.

The Seventh Day Adventists celebrate their Sabbath from sunset on Friday to sunset on Saturday. A twenty-four hour sanctuary in time, they call it.

9. THEY DRINK, BUT JUST A LITTLE BIT

These people drink a little bit every day, not a hard sell to the American people. Studies show drinking red wine reduces the risk of heart attacks and lowers stress.

While life expectancy is increasing around the world, recently it declined in the U.S. for the second year in a row.

When it comes to longevity, there is no short-term fix in a pill or anything else. When you think about it, your friends are long-term, and therefore perhaps the most significant thing you can do to add more years to your life and life to your years is spend time with them.

APPENDIX II

LITTLE THINGS THAT MATTER

(some of which doctors and other professionals may not know)

Recommended by the author of this book with input from the parties related to the topics.

For Caregivers:
DEMENTIA / ALZHEIMER'S PATIENTS

Some will keep fighting to walk out of the house, even in the heart of the night. Throw a black mat at the door entrance, and when they get there, they will see it like a big hole and be scared to cross over.

They remember issues of their lives dating many years back right to childhood better than recent events.

Avoid yelling when they act wrong because that makes them more aggressive. Instead invite them gently into a conversation, to the dinner table, into the bathroom, shower, the car, etc., if you want them to cooperate.

MISCHIEVOUS CLIENTS

Some pretend in mischief to be demented in an attempt to give you hard times. You should also be smart enough to detect that and be strict on them, so they don't abuse you.

HARMFUL TOOLS

Hide all knives and blades from Alzheimer's/ dementia patients and from those with autism. Many have often tried to harm themselves and caregivers or visitors with such tools.

TEMPERAMENTS

Take time to study the temperament of a client before you propose anything to her. Even those who are not affected by dementia have mood swings that can weigh heavily on the caregiver if she doesn't study the situation well to know how best to adapt.

PARKINSON'S PATIENT

These patients often have high fall risks, so always be very close to them especially when they are walking. Their tremors can sometimes be quite frightening, but just stay calm, stay close, and watch until she stops shaking. Then you will see her regain balance and continue her steps.

DIARRHEA & CONSTIPATION

Most times, the caregiver will find that the client is either constipating or having diarrhea. And they go drinking all sorts of medications to help out. That's not quite necessary because adjusting your feeding habit often solves the issue.

For the case of diarrhea, give them apple juice, some slices of white bread, and plain white rice and the diarrhea shall stop within a maximum of two days if there isn't infection. Avoid cake, ice cream, spinach and other green vegetables, high-fiber fruits, and milk for some days because these are all natural stool softeners.

Sometimes there is so much a do about a client not having a bowel movement for two or three days. Except it is going for more than two days that shouldn't be much cause for worry. Instead of swallowing all those pills to get a bowel movement, consume the foods mentioned that aren't good for diarrhea.

CHAIR-BOUND & BED-BOUND CLIENTS

Reposition them time and again. Turn the client to one side and place a pillow under one flap of her buttocks, up to her back, for light suspension. Then turn again after about two hours, repeating the process. That way, she will hardly develop sores.

BED & BUD SORES

Avoid letting the patient sit or lie on the position of the sore or it won't heal fast. Constantly apply a sore-healing cream.

STROKE PATIENTS

Regularly drink warm water heated on the stove or an electric kettle but not in the microwave. It helps blood circulation and dissolution of clots. Avoid cold water and cold foods. When consumed warm, they are more health boosting than cold food or cold water. Take a glass of warm water each morning and, if possible, with drops of lemon juice in it.

MASSAGE

The caregiver should give her client some massage frequently if she can. It facilitates blood circulation with good healing effects. Appropriate areas for that are the fingers, ankles, legs, feet, back, and corner of the neck and the back. This to be done very gently. You should massage the feet sliding upward to the knees, not the other way round.

WELL-KEPT HAIR AND NAILS

You will feel like some load is lifted off you when these two are taken care of, and especially when you wash your hair. It is recommended to do this weekly or every ten days if possible.

A caregiver is allowed to only file and not cut the nails of a client. These days, shampoo caps exist that can be used if you are bedbound and cannot go to the shower. Rinsing is not needed when this cap is used. It washes your hair quite clean, especially when it's not too thick. The cap is mostly ordered online, but it could be found in stores.

MUSIC

Play some soul-searching sounds that can keep your client away from the TV for a while and encourage singing of songs that both of you know.

EXERCISE

Take a walk down the block or street if you can rather than sitting indoors all day. It builds your immunity and is refreshing to the spirit and mind.

GARDENING

If the client has a small garden, always find time to do something there with her. The therapeutic effects on you both cannot be overemphasized.

PHONE ETIQUETTE

Use your phone only for essential calls while at work. Don't talk too loud to disturb the tranquility of the client.

EAT TOGETHER

Organize yourself to take your breakfast, lunch, and dinner at the time the client is having hers. That attracts patients with low or no appetite to eat.

SET ALARM

Set an alarm to remind you and your client of important things you have to do, like medication intake, if you cannot remember the care plan. Or write what is to be done daily on a blank, visible sheet and stick it where your eyes often look as you move around the house.

FALL RISK

When a fragile patient falls, never try to pick him up by yourself if he is heavy for you. That may cause him more harm. Call for help from a neighbor or an emergency unit.

Be always close and vigilant when with a client who is a fall risk, because their falls can easily cause damages beyond repair.

WHEELCHAIR

A client in a wheelchair should never be pushed with force because that could land her on the floor with her face first, resulting in a broken head and brain injury. When on an elevated spot, always pull the chair from the back. That means moving forward with her, with your face facing her back.

For Clients, Your Own Care :
BALANCED DIET

Having balanced diets frequently, that is, taking near equal portions of fruits, vegetables, and carbohydrates, upset bowels with diarrhea or constipation will likely become history to you.

SLEEP

Try to respect the scientifically recommended eight hour a night sleep, which gives you some essential vitamins that cannot be gotten from day sleep.

BEDDING

If you can change your bed sheets every week, you will find yourself sleeping quite deep each time that is done.

GAMES

If you have games and puzzles, play them because they keep your brain alert.

WHILE SITTING

Do some exercises as often as you can by just stretching out your feet, hands, neck, fingers, and other parts of your body. That saves you from stiffness and fat accumulation in your body. Don't always wait on the physical therapist to come assist you with that. Work it out with your aide.

RECLINING CHAIR

Very relaxing and relieving for the elderly and those having problems with their legs and knees. If you can afford one for your parent, don't hesitate. It's the best gift! It helps them stretch out their legs and eases circulation for those with water accumulating in them.

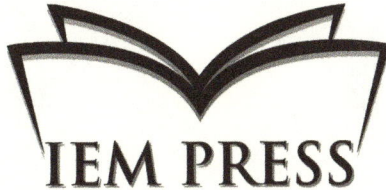

www.ingramcontent.com/pod-product-compliance
Lightning Source LLC
Chambersburg PA
CBHW030109300326
41934CB00033B/453